MASTERING HEALTH

THE IMPORTANCE OF THE MIND BODY CONNECTIONS

HOW TO MAINTAIN A HEALTHY LIFE

VERONIKA WINBANN O'NEILL

CONTENTS

INTRODUCTION

Most individuals are unaware of the fact that our minds and our body are directly connected. All that our body does is the product of commands provided by our brains. These commands are processed in many stages and cause many alterations that eventually make our body behave the way it does. Inversely, our body also influences our minds. The body is full of nerve endings that transmit messages to the brain. On receiving these messages, the brain responds. Even our internal organs are controlled by the brain, and they also send signals to the brain; it's on this basis that the brain delivers signals to the organs to react accordingly.

Therefore, to maintain a healthy mind, it is necessary to keep a healthy body, including internal organs, and vice versa. The more we shape our bodies, the more we shape our minds. Physical fitness is highly advantageous in this respect. Optimum physical activity helps to maintain a healthy body, both externally and internally, by controlling blood flow, increasing the oxygen-carrying ability of the blood, keeping the various parts and organs active, removing toxins from the body, and handling other biological processes that occur within the human body.

A healthy body battles many anomalies and manages to rejuvenate various sections and organs. This causes the brain to be at ease because a lot fewer stress messages are sent to it. Thus, a balanced body helps you develop independently with a quiet, balanced, and optimistic mind.

A balanced, optimistic mind is highly beneficial. Much as a healthy body could do more physical work, a healthy mind could do more mental work. Toxins that degrade the working capacity of the mind are not restricted to stress signals transmitted by the body. It also includes mental stress and disruptions, which, in turn, disturb the balance needed to maintain a safe and active mind.

The mind with chemicals, in the form of stress signals and other negatives that impair its working, functions less effectively and gets exhausted quickly. If all these toxins are removed as soon as they appear, the productivity of the mind improves. It gets tired less quickly, too. The brain works sharper and seeks both smarter and healthier solutions to all problems. It's more imaginative and profitable, too. In addition to this, a balanced mind tends to improve one's memory, improving your power of recollection.

CHAPTER:1

POSITIVITY CREATES THE WELLBEING THAT AFFECTS OUR ALL HUMAN COMPONENTS

WHAT IS WELLBEING?

Although there are many definitions of wellbeing, the fact that it is essential to everyone is indisputable. Well-being has many elements, such as mental, psychological, social, emotional, and spiritual dimensions.

- Social wellbeing is a feeling of belonging to a culture and a commitment to society.

- Emotional wellbeing means feeling healthy. To be happy, to experience positive emotions such as love, joy, or sympathy, and to feel generally pleased with life.

- Spiritual wellbeing can involve feeling linked to higher energy, a sense of meaning or reason, or a feeling of harmony or enlightenment.

Wellbeing can be defined as encouraging people to grow their abilities, to perform effectively and creatively, to build positive relationships with each other, and to make a meaningful contribution to the community.

There is a broader kind of wellbeing that comprises living in a way that is beneficial for you and good for those around you. Some other definitions of wellbeing include:

- Feelings of satisfaction, contentment, pleasure, interest, and loyalty to their society are the attributes of someone who has a good experience of their life.

- Equally significant for wellbeing is our ability to work well mentally in the world. Maintaining good relationships, getting some influence over one's life, and a sense of intent, self-esteem, and self-confidence.

- Wellbeing does not mean that you never encounter emotions or circumstances that are unpleasant for you, but it does mean that you believe that you can cope with stressful times.

Physical Well-Being
Improves cardiac functions, reduces hypertension, balances hormonal regulation., improves respiratory functioning, enhances eyesight.

Social Well-Being
Effective interpersonal communication, stronger bonds, deeper emotional attachment, empathy, less conflict and aggression at home.

Human-Nature Connection

Psychological Well-Being
Emotional regulation, increased attention, positive thinking, improved stress management, resilience, mood upliftment.

Spiritual Well-Being
Deeper sense of self, more gratitude, Self-enhancement, increased insight towards the positive and negative aspects of life.

It's important to remember that well-being' or wellbeing' is what you do, rather than what you are. The stuff we do and the way we feel can have a considerable effect on our lives.

Getting a positive attitude does not mean that you never have negative feelings, such as depression or anger. Both emotions - positive or negative - are adaptive in the right conditions. The key is to be to create a balance between the two.

Positive emotions broaden our consciousness and open up new ideas so that we can evolve and add to our survival toolbox. But people need negative feelings to move through challenging circumstances and respond effectively in the short term. Negative emotions can get us into difficulties, if they're focused on the past, spent speculating excessively about the future, and they're detached from what's going on here and now.

Experts claim emotionally healthy people, have less negative feelings, and can bounce back from setbacks faster. This quality is known as resilience. Another indication of mental wellbeing is being able to hang on to positive feelings longer and enjoy good times. Developing a sense of meaning and intent in life - and reflecting on what is important to you - also leads to emotional wellbeing.

Research has shown a correlation between an upturn in mental wellbeing and better health, including lower blood pressure, decreased risk of heart disease, healthy weight, improved blood sugar levels, and longer lifespan. However, several studies cannot determine if positive emotions contribute to improved health, whether being healthy induces positive emotions, or whether other factors are involved.

Previous research indicates a correlation between positive emotions and health, it does not disclose the underlying mechanisms. To understand the processes, I think it would be important to understand the underlying brain circuits.

Individuals that can enjoy positive feelings have long-lasting activation in the ventral striatum. The longer the activation lasts, the greater his or her feeling of wellbeing. Continued stimulation of this portion of the brain has been associated with healthier changes in the body, including lower levels of stress hormones.

Negative feelings, on the other hand, can activate the brain region known as the amygdala, which plays a role in fear and anxiety. Studies have shown significant variations between people in how quickly or slowly the amygdala recovers after the subject experiences danger. Those that recover more slowly could be at higher risk for a range of health problems compared to those who recover more rapidly.

People who practice different forms of meditation are among those who seem more resilient and better capable of holding on to positive emotions. In reality, increasing evidence indicates that a variety of techniques - including meditation, cognitive behavioral therapy (a form of psychotherapy), and self-reflection (appraising your thoughts and actions)-may help people develop the skills required to make meaningful, healthier changes.

Research points to the significance of some forms of training that can change brain circuits in a way that encourages positive reactions. It has led us to believe that wellbeing can be labeled as harnessing life skills. In fact, if you practice, you can get better at it.

BENEFITS OF WELL-BEING

Thousands of research studies have shown that wellbeing doesn't just feel good – it's vital for a happier, healthier lifestyle:

1. Optimism and optimistic thoughts can minimize the risk of a heart attack by up to 50%. Optimism can be practiced.
2. Experiencing three times more positive feelings than negative ones brings you to point where you become much more immune to adversity and better equipped to accomplish tasks.
3. Happier people live longer.

4. Our display of positive feelings, such as happiness and optimism, affects the people we meet, and studies show that our positivity can be transferred on to others.

5. High levels of wellbeing have been shown to improve our immunity to infection, reduce our risk of particular mental health issues, reduce mental deterioration as we grow older, and improve our resilience.

6. High levels of wellbeing are just as good for heart health and have as much protection from heart disease.

Research also shows that people who report higher levels of wellbeing appear to:

- Participate more in social events and community organizations
- Be ecologically conscious
- Experience healthier family and social interactions at home
- Be more efficient in the workplace
- Be more likely to engage in full-time employment or studying
- Be more likely to recover rapidly from a variety of chronic conditions (e.g., diabetes) and
- Show less likelihood of being hooked on alcohol, tobacco, and cannabis use.

CHAPTER:2

CREATE HEALTHY HABITS, NOT RESTRICTIONS

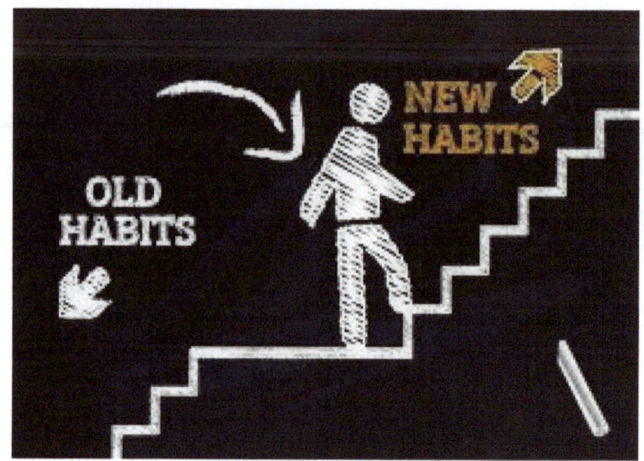

Being healthy doesn't mean that you should cut or limit things that you enjoy. It's all about lifestyle alterations that are going to be better for you. Don't be punished by way of limitations, but change your habit and see your improvement.

1. UNDERSTAND THAT VIBRANT WELLBEING STARTS FROM INSIDE

We all want to live healthy and be happy forever, and only a handful of us really live such a blessed life. Many define a healthy and happy human as a blessed individual. Achieving a healthy mind and body isn't really a blessing; it is the product of daily commitment and hard work to be the happiest and healthiest version of yourself implementing vital habits and good nutrition.

'You are just what you eat' – a term that justifies many inquiries by people eager to have a balanced body and mind. At present, as most of us are hooked to many unhealthful habits due to an increasingly busy lifestyle, the simplest definition of healthy living has become an art. Despite being open to a plethora of safe living tips and insightful material on the Internet, these days, people have miserably failed to achieve healthy lifestyles and eating habits. There needs to be a clearer understanding of the principle –Healthy outside begins from inside.'

Undoubtedly, most of us lack discipline in keeping a successful and safe regimen and are always moaning about being vulnerable to many health issues. How could a body with very poor health habits or, in fact, no healthy habits and no eating practice contribute to a healthy mind?

An unhealthy person can rarely be seen to be happy, and happiness often tallies with good health along with other life aspirations. And since health is the only wealth that leads to happiness and a productive life, why not start with easy steps towards a healthier life?

Definitely, we can make a ton of improvements in the way we've been unhealthy and miserable by practicing these good habits.

Here is the way to get started

1. Little Workout to Improve Immunity and Happiness

Practicing daily is one of the easiest ways to give the body and mind a vital boost. In reality, exercise is often seen as a remedy to keeping stress, unhappiness, and unhealthiness at bay. Not only can people with daily exercise activities maintain a healthy body, but they also improve their bod'y immunity and a feeling of satisfaction or contentment. It is because exercise helps the body release endorphin that reduces pain and raises the sense of joy and happiness. So, go out for a jog or begin to work with a 10-minute program on your cell phone, at least start exercising regularly.

2. Nourish Your Stomach With Healthy Foods

Do you know a chemical called serotonin found in our body that promotes a sense of happiness? 90% of the serotonin chemical is produced in our intestines. All we put in our stomach, therefore, affects our mood. Considering this crucial reality, include in your diet foods rich in nutrients and other health benefits. Make sure you stay away from refined foods, high sugar foods, repeated antibiotics, and starch diets. Practicing exercise, exercising daily, and removing negative self-talk or negative people from your life can alleviate tension are other things that bring worry and stress.

3. Always Stay Hydrated

Adequate consumption of water is a good routine that helps the body release and hydrate toxins quickly. It also improves kidney work and cleans the skin from inside. Also, balanced water consumption habit helps to strengthen the immune system and reduce fatigue. If plain water always seems drab and too routine, the squeeze in a lemon, add some sprig of herbs will make it beautiful-your body would certainly thank you for taking the right fluids.

4. Uncover Peace of Mind

If you have no idea how to achieve peace of mind, then you have to make a shortlist of everything you respect and want to see if you're really working towards it. Do you care about the small stuff or goal completion? Are you highly overscheduled? Is there something you're still thinking about? Now take a look at all your day-to-day problems and try to get rid of your fears about better options and invest extra time on things that give you a sense of satisfaction, like playing some sport, giving some time to your hobbies, speaking to people you love, and more.

4. Never Miss Your Breakfast

Breakfast is the most important meal of the day since it is the first meal you have after a long night of starvation. So, kicking off your day with a healthy meal such as eggs, rice, brown bread, organic fruit/vegetable smoothies, cereals, and others are a fantastic source of nutrients. These foods are absorbed rapidly by the body when you consume them in the morning as breakfast. Taking a decent amount of protein and avoiding unprocessed carbohydrates are great ways to manage body weight gain and reduce cholesterol levels. Eating breakfast every day without failing helps to restore glycogen and insulin levels in the body that make people feel less hungry, sick, and tired.

5. Take Proper Sleep

People who are either deprived of sleep or who do not have enough sleep are vulnerable to many health problems. Apart from always being in a bad/sick mood and feeling tired regularly, sleep-deprived people have bad digestion and low immunity. According to reports, short sleepers are often at a higher risk of heart attack or stroke than those who sleep for 7 to 8 hours every night. In addition, having enough sleep is an effective way to maximize your ability to focus, thereby boosting your efficiency at work.

6. Avoid Making Comparisons With Others

One of the most common ways people destroy their happiness is through a feeling of dissatisfaction borne out of comparing the results in their lives with those achieved by others. By having some kind of contrast with the lives of others, we put ourselves in a state of sadness. Such a sense of dissatisfaction and depression can reduce trust and make a person unhappy with their life, body type, achievements, and much more. Instead, strive to be satisfied and happy with what you have and work hard towards your well-thought goals.

Health is wealth, and being safe outside begins from the inside. So, every attempt should been made to follow good habits that can bring satisfaction; otherwise, life is too short to live miserably and unhealthy.

2: Establish Your Health Baseline Goals

The second step in taking care of your wellbeing is to set targets, and the "baseline" of your wellbeing is a smart way to do this. Gather some simple details that clearly inform you about your body weight, height, family background, exercise habits, general diet, and self-assessment of your stress levels at work and at home.

Some experts would incorporate medical tests that only a medical practitioner can administer, such as blood pressure, cholesterol and other lipids, and bone density. The difficulty with these assessments is that they allow you to fear. Being anxious is a poor motivator for the most people. It will keep you alarmed, in this state, people tend to give in to their fears, make terrible decisions, and raise their own stress levels. With that in mind, I'm going against the grain of conventional medical advice, at least in part, by saying that heeding these medical indicators should come second after you've been on a successful wellness program for at least six months. Offer consciousness a chance to kill it with possible anxiety.

How are you really setting your goals? Start thinking about this big picture. With the right support, changing poor lifestyle habits becomes easy, particularly if the challenge for you is smoking or overeating. To succeed, you need a clear vision of what you want to accomplish.

3: SET YOUR PRIORITIES

Making lists of your sad spots and happy spots will help you to set your personal goals. The sad spots are weaknesses, the happy spots are strengths that come to the fore with little effort. You can't get rid of every poor habit at once; it's nice to win a series of small victories at first.

Sad spots: list the moments you feel dissatisfied or most agitated - fighting a futile battle to get a decent night's sleep, maybe, or criticizing yourself for ordering dessert when you're already satiated. Identify the most significant problems with simple goals, such as going to bed on time, reducing food servings, avoiding candy, preferring a sofa over a treadmill, and so on. Doing this is going to help your purpose take shape and direction.

Happy spots: list the things that give you pleasure and happiness, such as spending time with friends and family or enjoying a favorite hobby. Recapture in your mind what it feels like to stop ordering dessert or spending half an hour walking outside. Appreciating the happy spots of your life is a source of power when you embark on your habit-changing quest.

4: DETECTING HARMFUL BEHAVIORS

You need to know what they are to improve your bad habits. Some poor habits, such as smoking and heavy drinking, are evident, but others may be less. Sitting all day is detrimental to your health, even though you have half an hour of exercise or more before or after work. Preventing yourself from eight hours of sleep for even a short period is often problematic for the body.

Forming a new habit requires practice and concentration, and if your attention is elsewhere, you can have a hard time adapting to new routines. For this reason, some experts warn against preparing drastic changes if you're going through an incredibly stressful time. I think the logic is incorrect. While it is true that you are likely to experience more relapses at times like these, it is just as true that people are improving as a result of overcoming obstacles and crises: -Aha moments happen very frequently when someone hits bottom.

Visualizing the ideal result is a valuable method for the path. "Seeing" yourself as you wish helped smokers quit, obese people lose weight, and sports champions accomplish their goals. To alter the body's printout, you must learn to rewrite the mind's program. This is supported by brain scans that show a decline in some higher functions (making right decisions, pursuing an urge over an another, and resisting temptation), when a person falls into a pattern of giving in to a broad range of lower urges, such as fear, rage, or simply physical hunger.

You need to apply a calming regimen that promotes and rewards your good decisions if you want brain pathways to follow suit.

5: MAKE A STEADY TRANSITION

Even if you're working on a big picture, a series of small wins is desirable for psychological reasons. Essentially, you train the brain to succeed. Most of us, having been defeated by old conditioning, follow the route of least resistance, not understanding that we train our brains on pathways that deprive us of free will over time.

So start with a victory that you can define, and that means something to you. Miss the red meat for one week. Take the stairs and not the lift. If you're out of shape, walk 10 minutes a day and gradually build up your time. Put your fork down halfway through your meal, take a few deep breaths, and ask yourself if you're still hungry. If you're sitting at a desk, make it a rule to always stand or walk while you're on the call. Over time, what seems to be baby steps induces new physiological changes in every cell of the body. Millions of cells listen to your every thought and action.

Rather than pretending that your body doesn't recognize what you're doing, offer yourself the gift of bringing good news to your cells.

However, in my opinion, the most significant victories are in awareness. If you appear to procrastinate, be mindful of the reasons for doing so. We're comfortable in our wet, cozy old routines, and making changes, even minor ones, feels psychologically threatening, as if even a positive change is a danger. Predict when you're going to procrastinate and invent a plan to deal with such a decision.

6: REINFORCE GOOD DECISIONS

Brain science also underlines the obvious, but it is a breakthrough to watch MRI scans and see for yourself that good actions' light up the brain in ways distinct from poor decisions. In the greater scheme, as you pursue a wellness program, every day, you will be faced with the option of staying in the course or abandoning your task. How does your mind make choices, then?

Executive control, which means choosing a thought or behavior to accomplish an internal purpose, is controlled by the prefrontal cortex of the brain. The orbitofrontal cortex and amygdala play a part in controlling decision-making based on the memory of emotions. The midbrain regions in which the neurotransmitter dopamine predominates often affects decision-making. Any decision that causes the release of dopamine: consuming sweet food, taking medications, having sex.

We might be over-indulged in chocolate cakes because we prioritize the short-term result we know (deliciousness) over the long-term result we have never experienced (losing weight and improved health from good nutrition). One way to escape this loop is to reward ourselves in a particular way. Instead of eating a cake, we should play a game or watch movies.

CHAPTER:3

BELIEVE YOU CAN, AND YOU'RE ALMOST THERE

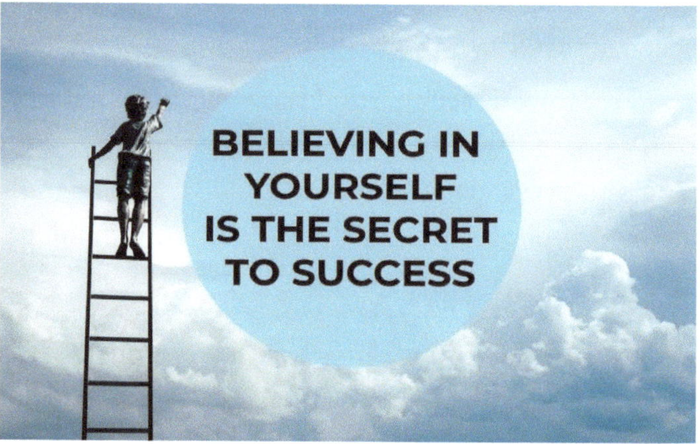

Believing in yourself will open up endless opportunities in your life. You may find it extremely difficult to do at times. The truth is that we've been habituated to doubt ourselves all our lives. We need to retrain ourselves to get rid of our worries and self-doubt to create self-esteem and self-confidence. Whatever you have in your life is the outcome of your belief in yourself and the certainty that this is possible.

To believe in yourself means having faith in your own abilities. It means knowing that you can do something - that it's beyond your capabilities. If you believe in yourself, you will conquer self-doubt and have the courage to take action and do things.

When you drown in fear, doubt, and self-sabotaging actions, success is beyond your reach. All of the world's skills, preparation, and resources won't change your life. If you solidify your confidence in yourself, you will achieve 100 % success.

1. FOCUS ON YOUR STRENGTHS (NOT YOUR WEAKNESSES)

When you struggle over and over in an area that seems straightforward to everyone, it's almost difficult to believe in yourself. Struggling with confidence, you prefer to concentrate on the stuff you can't do. That's how you sense vulnerabilities more closely.

You need to know how to define your strengths, so you can make the most of the mileage out of them. A common practice of successful people is to concentrate on the positive - what they succeed at - and to assign failures to others instead of thinking about not measuring up. When you turn your attention to cultivating your strengths, you can feel more capable and confident effortlessly.

Knowing your strengths will encourage you to bring more focus into places where you're already talented. You should evolve in the way that you are naturally inclined. Once you operate based on courage and confidence in your skill, you can find the motivation to do something about it.

Recognizing your innate talents (and inability) gives you permission to avoid bashing your head against a wall. You should do what you do best and find workarounds for the rest of the time.

For example, starting a company requires a lot of skills, but you don't have to own all of them:

- You're great at ads, but you're bad with numbers. Outsource your accounting and employ a specialist to handle your budget.

- You shine on creating content, but you're afraid of engaging with social media. Using automation software to handle part of your work or employ a strategist.
- You enjoy preparing a big picture, but get lost when it's time to execute it. Take a partner who can get the project off the ground.

Use your power to your advantage. This method will give you confidence while you concentrate on using your best skills. Shifting everything else off your plate gives you the ability to be excellent at what you do best.

Your talents make you unique. Develop and depend on these qualities.

2. Be A Mentor Of Your Own

If you don't believe in yourself, you're not going to believe someone who cheers you from the sidelines. Great coaches and administrators inspire people to succeed with the right tools, education, and opportunities to become outstanding. They connect with people using methods like Conversational Intelligence to make people feel relaxed and bring out the best of everyone.

Research demonstrates that positive thinking, target setting, and performance evaluations do not yield results independently. If you don't believe you've got what it takes, none of that stuff is a magic bullet. So how do you make the most of this experience and prepare yourself?

Find the resources and resources you need to grow your talent. Take action now. Every move you take, getting closer to your target, is proof of your ability to succeed. Believing in yourself will be simpler and simpler the more you see your progress mirrored back to you.

The secret is, there's no need for another person to work through this process. You don't need to have the skills of leadership to train yourself through it. The key is to think more about yourself without becoming a judge.

Start by writing where you want to be in your life. Write down all the things you want to have, and the kind of person you want to be. You can come up with strategies from this to get to that point. What does success look like to you?

Choosing ideas that suit you - and working with your strengths - may lead you to your own vision of success. You should even write down the aspects of your life that you're dissatisfied with. Create action and find the tools to develop all of these areas:

- Feeling overwhelmed by duty
- Want more meaning in life
- Want more free time for things you enjoy (reading, gardening, hiking)
- Financial burden

By recognizing the areas of your life that you are least pleased with and keeping an eye on where you really want to be, build long-term goals that are achievable for you. Set a large target at a time, then break it down into smaller pieces. Performance in taking any small step into action, no matter how small, leads to noticeable change. At the end of the day, these persistent small achievements lead to self-confidence and huge trust. With time, you're starting to see that you can do everything you're dreaming about - because you're already doing it.

3. EMBRACE WHO YOU ARE

How do you believe in yourself when you don't know who you really are? Or worse, you're trying hard to be someone you're not. Self-confidence comes from accepting who you are and what is important to you. It doesn't come from being genuine or trying to impress people. The pressure to fit in, to "be natural," is high, and starts early. That's all right if you want to live an unremarkable life. But you're here to read this post because it's no life for you. You like a bit more.

To start believing that you can have the life you want, you have to dig deep to figure out what it's going to look like for you. You have to realize what makes you special and celebrate the stuff. When you begin to live true to your identity and core values, you start to believe in your worth, your capacity, and your human potential.

It's best to welcome yourself in baby steps:

a) Start By Writing Down What Is Important To You.

You're going to want to do this a few times over weeks or even months, and you get closer to uncovering your core values. This is going to make you see things that you've been programmed to believe in. When you're done, you're going to have a list of characteristics that reflect your truest self.

b) Observe Your Patterns Of Thinking And Actions.

Do you always take care of others at the detriment of your own values? If you think you're cool, or if you're still in peace, ask yourself why. The end result is that you dim your own shine and live for the praise of others.

When you sense this, an internal struggle is going on, try to fix it. You may kindly say no, make a different opinion, or let others know that what they did affected you. Maybe some people don't like the -new you, and that's okay. They may have a more limited role to play in your life. Luckily, when you are really you, the right people will be attracted to you, and real friendships will grow deeper.

c) Get Out Of The Standards Of Others.

Being authentic seems like a huge risk, and you may be afraid of being critical. Know that your life experience is about you, and their life experience is about you. Doing things that scare you will solidify the confidence you need to be your most authentic self. It sounds counter-intuitive, but being vulnerable - receiving your fear and not hiding it - is the surest road to building power.

Create time for adventures that are totally out of your daily routine. It could be jumping out of a plane, taking a workout class, or taking a paintbrush. Choose something that seems interesting, but you're scared at least a little bit and jump in. You will learn so much about yourself from these experiences that you can take part in them regularly. Bring variety and sometimes do new things.

4. Believe That You Will and You Can

Your conviction is the single most important weapon you've got. You can change your life absolutely only by changing your values. It's not wishful thinking - to imagine that anything affects how you see the world and yourself. Either you see opportunities, or you see insurmountable barriers. Who are you going to choose?

To start believing in yourself, you've got to stop thinking that you're stuck with the talents and abilities you have right now. This is called a fixed mind, which is a narrow pattern of thought that is lethal to your success. Instead, start believing that you can improve yourself. This way of thinking is called a mind of development. It means that you assume that progress is possible. It might be accurate that you don't have what it takes to reach your goals - right now. But if you believe that you can change, grow, and learn, you're going to get there - even if nothing's going right.

Firmly believing that you and your life will improve for the better is the driving force behind all your efforts. You will then be more eager and even more motivated to get the work you need to do to make those improvements. There is no greater booster of trust than seeing the results of your work. But you have to believe it's worth it, or you're never going to make an attempt.

5. Be uncomfortable

If what you did today looks a lot like what you did yesterday, last week, and three years ago - you're too relaxed. You're in a pattern, and it just doesn't get you anywhere. You have to get uncomfortable to make a meaningful difference in your life. You've got to get out of your comfortable box and do things differently.

This means making more effort, and even feeling a little odd, to do things that are out of the ordinary. You've got this whole life to play with who you are. It's your life, and you don't have to live it to meet the demands of someone but your own. If you want to have a different life, make it yourself. By experimenting and acting on your thoughts, your strengths and ability are mirrored back to you.

Experience with various abilities, techniques, and strategies in your life is one of the best ways to build trust and cultivate mental strength. Sure, this is awkward! There are always new things. Luckily, when you start to do more new stuff, fear becomes fun. You learn so much by trying new stuff, whether or not you succeed in the attempt.

There are problems here. Part of the process includes getting over negative self-talk, fear of failure, and imposter syndrome. You can have to face real anxiety and figure out ways to handle it. Every single person who has made some kind of self-improvement can tell you that these feelings are genuine. They're going to tell you it's scary, but the results are worth it. There will be fear every time you walk into something different. Your strength is to walk through the fear and do the thing anyway.

Magic occurs simply by believing that this is possible. Your confidence in the possibility is essential for the work, the experimentation, and the discipline required changing your life. This belief in possibility is what has provided rock stars with single-minded intensity to get on stage every night, in the face of ludicrous odds.

It's what has given popular writers the tenacity to keep writing and editing despite several rejected manuscripts. It's what kept the star athletes practicing, through pain, injury, and loss, until they did it to the top. Now you've got some tools to start believing in yourself. Act on these steps regularly, and you'll begin to see incredible things happening in your life.

CHAPTER:4

YOU ARE WHAT YOU EAT, SO ALWAYS CHOOSE THE BEST

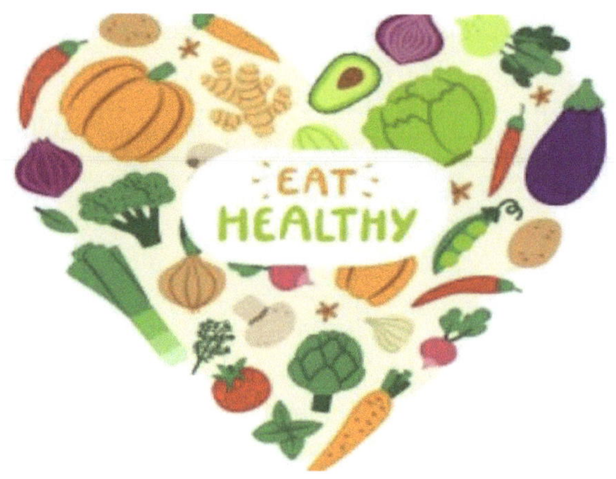

The planet is full of various dishes and tons of different meals. Even when we reduce them to their base, there are only a handful of ingredients that our bodies need to live. These simple molecules come from various classes we're all familiar with - carbohydrates, fat, protein - each type of molecule is significant for the way our bodies function. So, what to pick from?

Our physical and emotional wellbeing is directly related to what we are eating and drinking. The nutritional content of what we eat is determined by the composition of our cell membranes, bone marrow, blood, hormones, tissues, organs, skin, and hair. Every day, our bodies replace billions of cells - and use the food we eat as a source.

A well-balanced diet not only results in improved health and overall body composition but can also make us feel fantastic due to the -brain-gut relation. Eating healthy is part of a plan that can reduce the risk of chronic illness and even boost the condition of our own genes. There's no -o ne rule fits all when it comes to eating healthy. Applying the widely accepted guidelines, such as low sugar, low salt content, and a wide range of nutrients, could be the most advisable for all of us.

Giving attention to how much we consume is another very critical part of good nutrition - which inevitably affects all of us. What we eat and how much we eat is crucial, but it could be even more important to process it. Via thousands of small sensors, the intestine has the enormous task of handling all the information found in the food we consume. Food alone will not guarantee a flourishing intestine.

If you eat a healthy and delicious meal with a friend, but all of a sudden, you start battling each other - your stomach will shut down, and you will probably feel indigestion, discomfort, or nausea. And when we eat by ourselves, most of us have a constant internal conversation in our minds. We are packed with innumerable thoughts and feelings that draw all our attention from the food in front of us. We're also eating while on the phone, on the TV, and at our desk. There is reason to believe that eating when we are emotional, confused, or simply distracted can slow down or stop digestion.

When we experience extreme emotions, such as stress or anxiety, our usual, mechanical, intestinal digestive process - most of which operates independently - will be affected and altered. Stress hormones, such as adrenaline, norepinephrine, and cortisol, can communicate with the cells in our intestines, making us alert and ready to battle or travel. By paying attention to our mental state of eating, we will enhance our processing of food. Our body parts are related to our emotions, but the gut sends the strongest signal to our brain's emotional centers.

It can be as easy as being more conscious of the act of eating itself - including hearing, smelling, chewing, and swallowing. We may also expand our focus on the impact that food has on our bodies and our mood. Going even further, we can be regarded as the earth that gives us this driving force that we call food.

Researchers have actually found that teaching such -mindful eating skills will improve bad eating habits. Mindful eating trials have shown that participants dramatically reduced compulsive eating habits, enhanced self-control, decreased depressive symptoms, lost weight, and retained their weight loss for long periods.

By paying attention to all the nuances and layers of knowledge involved in our diet, we will also awaken our intestines - in turn, helping us make better decisions about the foods we consume and the quantities we consume in the future.

CHAPTER:5

THE BODY ACHIEVES WHAT THE MIND BELIEVES

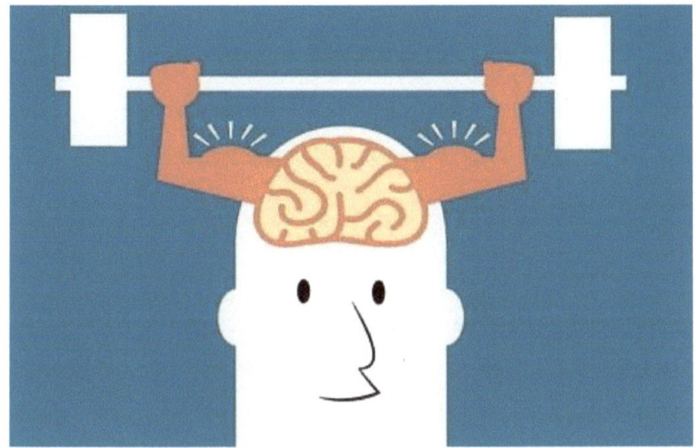

Believe in yourself, you can do anything you set your mind to do. There are no limitations out here; the only restrictions are those you put on yourself. Dream, trust and take action. Identify what you really want, how you really want to live your life, and take action. Start building the life of your dreams. Start tiny, dream big, and never give up.

You've got to go for what you want, or you're going to be confined to the life you've stumbled into. Most people are relegated to a life of mediocrity because they don't try to make a concerted effort searching for what their hearts desire. They just live their entire lives like cowards, afraid to get out of their comfort zone, but it's not even the comfort zone that people want to call it, it's the lazy zone, just getting through the area, the cowardice zone, the conformist zone.

You've got to know that there's something inside you, and that's greatness. Inside is where real growth is taking place that will allow you to live the life of your dreams. The mind is the key to unlocking the door to your potential, your fearlessness, your courage, your ambition, your drive, your determination, your hunger, your grit, your perseverance, and your greatness.

Do away with the mentality of mediocrity; you have to step up your game and take your life to a new level. Now is the time to go after what you really want, change your mind, and your life will begin to change. We don't see the world as it is, just as it is. When you change for the better, everything around you will change for the better. Your outside world represents your inner world.

If you don't believe that you can do something that you're aware of, it's because you have some incorrect internal assumptions about yourself. It's your conviction that determines how you live your life. If you don't believe that you can be good, then you're not going to do something, and you're just going to keep doing the same mediocre stuff day after day, and you're never going to chase after your dreams.

You're capable of more than you know, start improving yourself, start reprogramming your mind, and don't just settle for the so-called regular life. Most people are not going to work because they want to, because they have to pay their bills. Is that what the intention of the job is? You pay your bills? If it wasn't a matter of money, what would you do with your life? How would you like to live your life? What's your response to that? Everyone has an answer to that question, but the question is, what do you spend your days doing? Are you living a lie like most of the people?

It doesn't matter about your history, it doesn't matter how young or old you are, it doesn't matter how you did at school, it doesn't matter what you didn't do, and it doesn't matter how many mistakes you've faced. You can do something. Turn your page and rewrite a new story, don't let the first chapter of your life decide the rest of your life.

Forget the past, we've all had our fair share of life's disappointments, but don't live in the past; it's gone. So now, decide to be a new you, an individual who is determined to succeed and to live life on your terms. Make this day a new beginning for a new adventure of greatness. It's time to get on with your grind by focusing your mind on success.

It's the mind that keeps most people from going after what they really want. The mind is what paralyzes people to take action. Once you break down the mental barriers that have put you in jail, you will live life; differently; your perspective, your actions, your goals, your plans, your limits, and your fears will disappear.

I firmly believe that you can do whatever you set your mind to do. There's all the power inside of you to be whoever you want to be. Only you can restrict this ability. Don't let your worries determine the path you're going in your life. Do you believe that you can accomplish anything you want? Some people do, and they seem to be in a position to go for what they want and get it. While some struggle to satisfy their needs and seem to face dissatisfaction and disappointment.

They continue to come up short, no matter what they do. So is it really possible to do whatever you want in your life? Simply put, the two stories above, and many more tell us the answer is yes.' In our lives, we can do whatever we want. As long as we are committed to our goals and excited about our dreams, we will achieve them.

I believe that every person out there has their own unique passion that can motivate them to do whatever they really want. Alas, many of you won't force yourself out of your comfort zone and drop your pessimistic views, false perceptions, and sabotaging fears that have held you back to this point. But let's hope my blog makes a lot of you get up and go for it, at last. Can you think back to a point in your life when you first accomplished something? What a boost it gave to your confidence, and the rush of adrenaline carried you up to the stars.

At that point, you realized that you could do something if you really put the effort in. You still have the strength inside of you. Everyone has the power to do whatever you want. It's all about pushing you to the top! You can't wait to get inspiration. You've got to go after that with a club. Jack London Creativity will make things happen. When you're inspired, you're going to reach beyond what you were before. Your life is taking on a new vitality.

Know what's inspiring you. Look at what's missing in your life right now, so you can go for it. Commit to taking steps that will drive you out of your comfort zone and into new uncharted territories. Commit to your personal development and understand your potential. The will to win, the drive to succeed, the willingness to fulfill your full potential are the keys that will open the door to personal excellence.

STEP 1: KNOW WHAT YOU'RE LOOKING FOR

You've got to be crystal straightforward about what you want. Do not take the power of setting the target too lightly. Without targets, you won't stay focused on the direction you want to move; you'll be too easily distracted. You need to be explicit about the particular outcome you want to achieve and concentrate on that outcome.

STEP 2: KNOW WHY YOU WANT TO DO THAT

When you know what you really want, you need to understand why you want to do it – your goal of trying to achieve this outcome. Why would you like it? What's going to be different when you have it? How's life going to be better? When you know why you want it, you have a compelling reason that gives you the motivation to follow through, no matter what. The reasons come; first, the solutions come second. Your aim is to provide you with an emotional incentive to follow through and do whatever it takes to achieve the result you want.

STEP 3: FOCUSING ON YOUR DREAMS

Now that you know exactly what you want out of your life, you need to focus 100% on achieving it. When you put 100% emphasis on it, you'll certainly do whatever it takes to achieve it. When you concentrate on what is really most important to you in life, you will begin not only to achieve extraordinary results but most importantly, you will experience an unparalleled degree of personal satisfaction in the process.

STEP 4: STUDY, RESEARCH, AND ANALYSIS

If you're going to give everything you need to do something, make sure you know everything there is to know about it. Make yourself an expert in whatever area you choose to try. When you're an expert, you've got an advantage, and you'll feel more positive about going after your dream.

STEP 5: BUILD A STRATEGY FOR THIS.

What particular acts do you need to take to achieve this result? Write an action plan as a road map for your path towards your goals. When you embark on a journey to a new destination, you need a map to find your way. Make the strategy as comprehensive as possible, so there's no room for doubt. Your plan is simply a concrete phase or action that you need to take to achieve your result.

Step 6: Take Steps To Make This Happen.

Now that you've got a plan, you've got to put it into effect. Your dreams will remain unfulfilled until you begin to take steps to turn them into reality. You know, without taking steps, nothing is going to happen. You've got to fight for it; you've got to get the results. Still take massive action, no matter what you do. Taking action is going to build momentum. Take huge, continuous action.

Step 7: Trust Yourself And Your Goals.

You have to trust that you will accomplish your goals and that your dreams will come true. If you don't believe in what you do, you're never going to achieve what you want. Belief is what's driving you. You need to have a strong conviction before you can do anything about it. Believe that you will satisfy your wishes, and step in the direction of your beliefs. If you believe that you can, you can; if you don't think that you can, you can't. You can do that, just believe it!

Step 8: Be Totally Engaged.

To achieve incredible results in your life, you have to be 100 % dedicated, and you have to be willing to give your time and effort. This is where most of the people fall short. They lack a true sense of responsibility and are not able to invest their time taking targeted steps towards their goals. But the first thing you need to do is decide whether you're serious about your dreams and goals. It will take proper dedication and determination, and you must make the requisite hard work and effort.

Step 9: Keep Track Of Your Success.

As you take action and carry out your strategy, keep track of your progress. If you get results, keep doing what you're doing. If you don't see the impact then look at what you can alter. The person who is committed to bringing his life in a particular direction must always stop thinking and ask himself the question, -Is this going to lead me towards the goal I want to achieve?

STEP 10: DON'T GIVE UP

It won't be easy to achieve your target. Often things are going to get rough on your path. It's tempting to just give up, but if you don't struggle, you'll be cheating on yourself. Appreciate how far you've come and what you've done and know it's worth it. So, know what you want, build up your confidence that you want it so much that you'll be prepared to make a big effort, and be sure that your target will be achieved. Keep the drive in place, and make sure you remain committed to your goals and dreams.

CHAPTER:6

BECOME A PRIORITY IN YOUR OWN LIFE

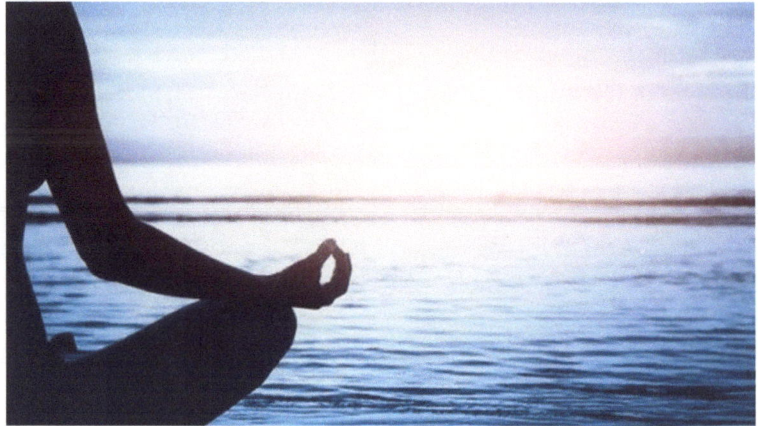

How would you be a better version of yourself? A blend of caring for both your mind and your body will get you there.

You know you want to go from the place 'I am here now,' to the zone 'This is where I wanted to be,' but you don't understand how. Yeah, you're not alone. Almost everybody else out there is going through the same problem. They work more than they live. As a life coach, I have learned that people want to conquer the fear of confronting themselves and understanding themselves; to recognize what is holding them back; to define their goal; to clear up the physical, emotional, and professional mess; or to deal with their distress with relative ease. Like you, everybody hopes that they will turn things around and improve for the better.

You could have been putting yourself in second place to something or another: a job, children, a loved one, popularity, wealth ... the list is endless. Maybe it's time to put yourself in the first place and do something about the difference between where you are right now and where you'd like to be.

You can start by taking care of yourself - of your mind, body, and soul.

SELF-CARE OF THE MIND

Make your priority to happiness. If you're not happy, there should be no one else around you. Delete or mute something that upsets you - people, feelings, trolls, and so on.

- Understand the way of thinking. Think about what works well and what doesn't; your principles and values; and use that knowledge to understand yourself.

- Indulge in specific self-reflection. Understand what and how you think about it. Be mindful of your thoughts and emotions.

- Focus inward. Be mindful of how you feel, what you need, and what you think at all times. This requires preparation, but it can be done really well. Know that this is like a tool, as you are still aware of what's going on inside you. Maybe that's the cherry on the cake when it comes to self-care.

- Laugh out loud. Don't be too serious; laugh at stuff. Watch or read something funny - anything at all, to laugh.

- Free for an hour. Switch off your phone for an hour and enjoy the ease that comes with not understanding it all.

SELF-CARE OF THE BODY

Find out what your body wants and try to produce. Learn to listen to the body and study it. It will help you give your body the right fuel (such as healthy food) to work and think quickly and clearly.

- Eat what you need, not what you want to eat. Poor food (e.g., fast food or thick, oily dishes) takes more time to digest, which ensures that you feel lethargic and need more sleep,

- Grow and shine every day. A few minutes of the sun's going to keep your body charged.

- Indulge in mindful exercise. Shift your body around. Exercise, run, walk, go up and down the stairs, enter a gym, do yoga, etc. Study to communicate with your body and become aware of its signals and signs. Pay attention to what you feel about it and deal through it. Your body has not been made to be sedentary.

- Respect and enjoy your body as it is. Look at your naked self in the mirror.

- Sleep well. Enable your body to have some much-needed rest.

SELF-CARE OF THE SOUL

Be very self-aware. Remove from yourself and become an observer. Reflect on your day every night, every day.

- Take care of your time. Your time is in your possession, but it is restricted. Use this wisely. If you're not interested or worth your time, it's not worth pursuing.

- Be a counselor and boss of your own. Tell yourself about the five Ws. When you're in trouble, ask yourself what it is, when it happens, where it happens, why it happens, and who makes it happen. Your answers are going to bring you to your own solutions. Check, too, what makes you happy at this moment; why do you feel amazing right now? Take care of yourself and learn how to be your own consultant in times of calm and chaos.

- You are an idol, too. Amid all your problems, you might forget that certain people around you look up to you, watch you and idolize you (your spouse, children, relatives, acquaintances, colleagues, and others). Only strive to be an ideal leader.

- Befriend yourself, man. Treat yourself once in a while. Do something self-nourishing. Do whatever you want - with yourself, alone.

- Be with the right people, give, and receive. Choose to be around people who have a positive effect on your life.

- Don't cling to what's done. What's over here is over; carry on.

- Be gentle with yourself, please. It takes time for anything, including transforming yourself to

- be the best version of you.

- Changing is the most successful way to start leading and living your life to the fullest. If you remember, the most important word here is leading.' You've got to lead your life, not let it show you to achieve what you want.

STUFF YOU SHOULD DO TO MAKE YOURSELF A TOP PRIORITY.

1. Please Make Time For You

It's not forgiving; it's okay to make time for you. However, you like to relax; putting aside some downtime to rest is vital to your wellbeing. Whether reading, diary, watching a movie, or taking a bath, take your foot off the pedal and find something that calms your mind and meets your needs.

2. Please Talk To Yourself

How many times did you find yourself thinking something terrible about yourself? Put an end to self-criticism and respond with sympathy to your concerns and uncertainties. If you don't say that to a friend, don't say that to yourself.

3. Get Rid Of The Iniquity

We spend so much of our time prioritizing the needs of others that we sometimes feel guilty or selfish when we decide instead to do something for ourselves. Change your mind and note that you don't need to justify taking care of yourself. Ever, ever.

4. Avoid Saying -Yes To All Of Them

It's easy to lose yourself in the -go, go, go attitude, but when you stop trying to satisfy others and do what you want to do instead, you're going to claim back so much happiness. Life is hectic, and you can't always ignore your own needs to meet someone else's needs. It's all right to feel the pleasure of losing out sometimes.

5. Loving The Skin That You're In

We're all guilty of dwelling on what we look like when we're supposed to admire our bodies for the extraordinary vehicle they are. They help us to breathe, to walk, and to love – they don't deserve this kind of criticism. Revel in the strengths of your body; celebrate the miles you can run or the child you've made. There's so much more to life than to think about imperfections.

6. Don't Be Afraid To Ask For The Support

You're just human, you have boundaries and limitations like anyone else, and you can't always do it on your own. Lean on your mates, ask what you want and what you need – there's pleasure in opening up and communicating with others.

7. Let Go Of Things That You Can't Control

Learn to let go of it! You can't influence the past, the future, or how other people see you, and the sooner you make peace with that, the happier you will be.

Why are we over-analyzing everything? Do we have to do it all perfectly all the time? Give yourself a little slack and stop punishing yourself for every misstep.

8. Tell Yourself That You Can

You can't banish the word; it doesn't exist in your vocabulary. Try new stuff, turn skepticism into belief - you're so much more capable than you know.

9. Embrace Your Feelings

Take the peaks with the pits and be kind to yourself in difficult times. Forcing yourself to get over something isn't making you deal with it any easier, relying on your feelings and allowing yourself to feel insecure when you need to. Your future self is going to thank you for that.

10. Surround Yourself With Some Good People

People who feel like sunshine are the keepers. Your friendships should raise you up, motivate, and empower you to develop as a person. It might sound heartless, but if you're no longer helping each other, there's no sense in trying to hang on to friendship when you can invest in someone who has a positive effect on your life. Friendship is not an unbreakable vow; if you lose your own happiness, it's more than okay to move on.

11. Start A Journal Of Gratitude

It might sound like it's one more thing to add to your to-do list every day, but starting a gratitude journal is a perfect way to focus on the here and now. It's a healthy habit to get into if you want to change your mind, forget about moaning, and concentrate on the joy of every day. Days and weeks in a flash, but pause to write about what you're grateful for, will make even the most meaningless days all the more memorable when you look back.

12. Know That You're Nice Enough

Appreciate how far you have come; your personal development and success is not something that needs to be brushed off. Acknowledge your wins and be so proud of yourself. There's no need to alter who you are to fit into someone else's definition of perfection; you don't need to prove anything to anyone. You're good enough because you're caring, you're good enough because you love intensely, you're good enough because you make others happy. Any part of you that already exists is what makes you good enough.

SUMMARY

The delivery of adequate and appropriate care to people with developmental disorders who have been active in the criminal justice system continues to pose significant obstacles to both the psychological health and criminal justice systems. Program initiatives have focused either on early diversion from the criminal justice system or on lowering the rate of recidivism. Jail diversion attempts, for example, have been made by mental health courts and drug courts to limit or slow down the admission of people with behavioral health problems into prison systems, and there is an increased focus on educating local police officers to properly handle their encounters with people with disruptive behaviors. On the other hand, a new wave of re-entry programs has tried to address the diverse needs of those made available to the community with little planning, training, or successful community programs.

Several state and local authorities have sponsored creating a specialized forensic peer specialist' workforce to meet the needs of either prison diversion or re-entry programming initiatives. This workforce is composed of people with a history of mental illness and/or imprisonment that have attained a reasonable sense of stability in their own lives and are now appointed by local government and non-profit organizations to provide individualized care to those with psychological disorders in criminal justice.

Forensic peer specialists (FPSs) are also operating on a one-on-one basis with referrals from mental health and substance abuse courts to provide previously inaccessible ongoing assistance that users might require to prevent incarceration in the future. A few FPSs work with individuals inside prisons and jails to develop re-entry policies to ensure a seamless transition to community life. However, most FPSs operate through community-based re-entry services to provide personal support and practical assistance in the months following release. The FPS sector is still very new, with work requirements and job responsibilities variously specified from site to site, funding cobbled together from various sources, and, most of the time, evaluation research.

Right now, powered by Ideological and financial imperatives, the workforce of the FPS is expected to grow in the future. The aim of this Policy Brief is to identify what we currently know about this new workforce and to set a research plan for the future.

After a decade or more of work in the field of mental health, the FPS sector developed Certified Peer Specialists' as a crucial and fundable factor in the delivery of community mental health resources. The National Mental Health Customer Empowerment argues that many other social care systems have benefited from focusing on individuals with their own experience of challenges to provide assistance to someone like themselves. From human services users, individuals who have been there,' they claim, are more readily trusted, more likely to understand and sympathies with one's concerns, and also better able to act as guides and advocates.

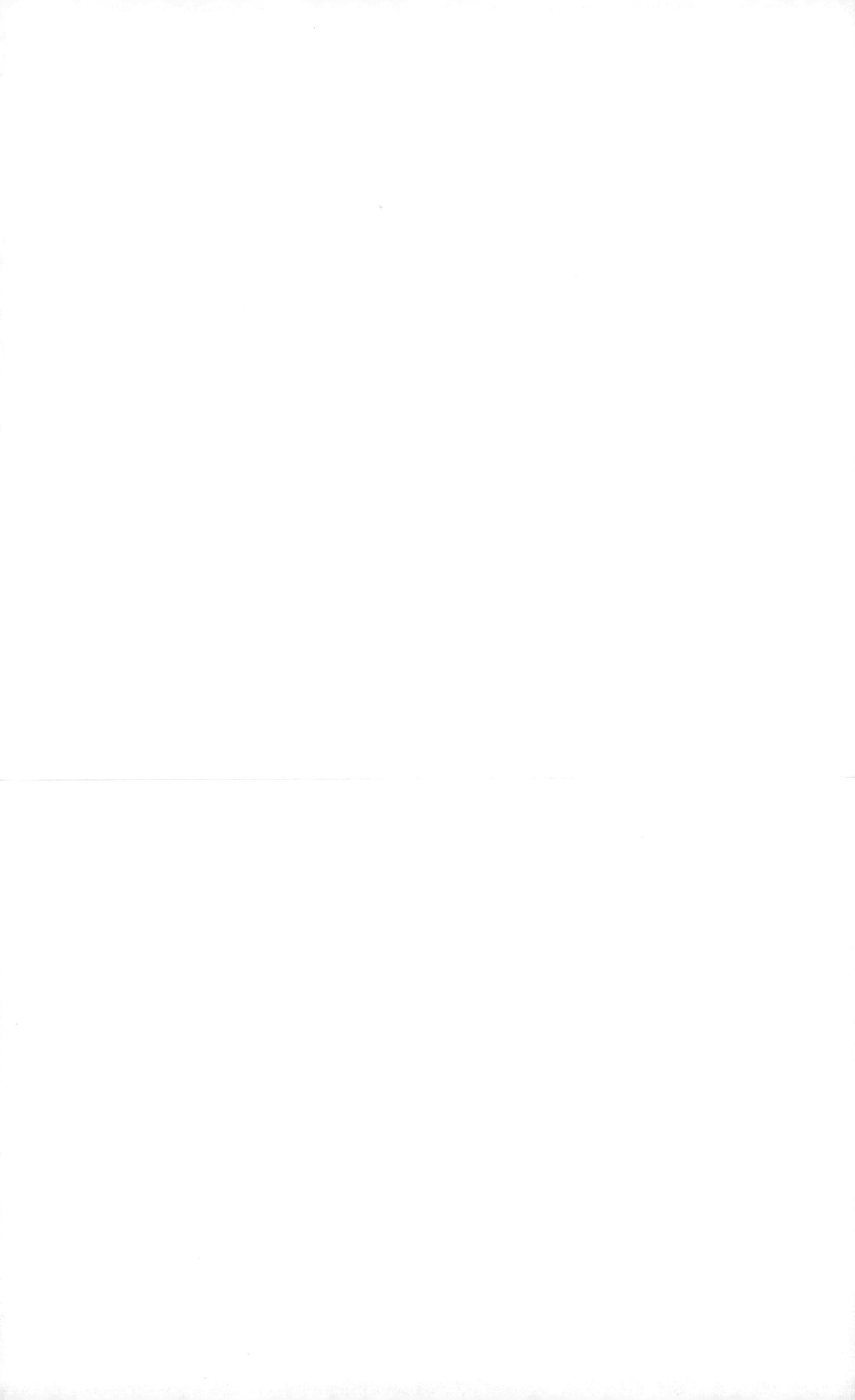